A HANDBOOK OF
CONSTRICTIVE PERICARDITIS
— AND —
ENDOMYOCARDIAL FIBROSIS

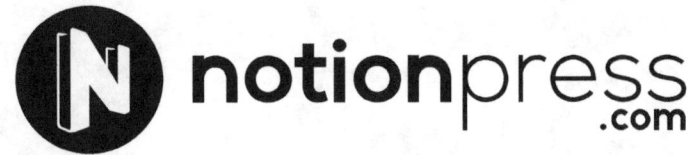

A HANDBOOK OF
CONSTRICTIVE PERICARDITIS
AND
ENDOMYOCARDIAL FIBROSIS

Monograph on Constrictive pericarditis
and Endomyocardial fibrosis

DR. ALOK RANJAN

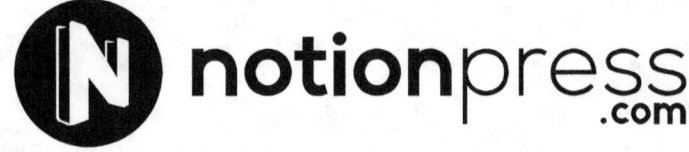

Notion Press

Old No. 38, New No. 6
McNichols Road, Chetpet
Chennai - 600 031

First Published by Notion Press 2017
Copyright © Dr. Alok Ranjan 2017
All Rights Reserved.

ISBN-10:1946641855

Paperback: 978-1-946641-85-4

Hardcase: 978-1-946641-88-5

Disclaimer

Medicine is a constantly changing science. New research findings necessitate continual changes in disease concept and its management. The author and publisher of this handbook have used reasonable efforts to provide up-to-date, accurate information that is within generally accepted medical standards at the time of publication. However, as medical science is ever evolving, and human error is always possible, the author and publisher (or any other involved parties) do not guarantee total accuracy or comprehensiveness of the information in this handbook, and they are not responsible for omissions, errors, or the results of using this information. The reader should confirm the accuracy of the information in this handbook from other sources. In particular, all drug doses, indications, and contraindications should be confirmed in package inserts.

The author has made every effort to trace the copyright holders for borrowed material. If he has inadvertently overlooked any, he will be pleased to make necessary arrangement at the first opportunity.

Dedication

Dedicated to my teachers and friends at KEM Hospital, Mumbai, Maharashtra, India

"It is commonly said that a teacher fails if he has not been surpassed by his students. There has been no failure on our part in this regard considering how far they have gone."

Edmond H. Fischer

Table of Contents

Constrictive Pericarditis

Constrictive Pericarditis (CP)

Introduction

Pericardium: Normal thickness is less than 3 mm (1.2 ± 0.8 mm) and the normal fluid content between the 2 layers is less than 50 ml (usually 10-20 ml). The pericardium limits the position and motion of the heart, limits dilatation and provides a barrier to the spread of disease from the lungs. Pericardium covers not only the heart but the fibrous layers are reflected at least by 10 mm over pulmonary veins, aorta, SVC and IVC. IVC has the least pericardial reflection among the great vessels. At least one hepatic vein ends very close to IVC – RA junction, thus likely to be involved in pericardial disease.

Association of characteristic hemodynamic changes and abnormal pericardial thickness > 3 mm usually confirms the diagnosis of constrictive pericarditis.

Constrictive pericarditis can be defined as a syndrome (or syndromes) resulting from compression of the heart caused by rigid, thickened and frequently fused pericardial membranes.

Constrictive pericarditis should be suspected in all patients with findings suggestive of right heart failure or ascites; diagnosis is usually not difficult provided there is an adequate index of suspicion.

Diagnosis should be based on a triad of a suggestive clinical syndrome, demonstration of a physiology of constriction/restriction and demonstration of a thickened pericardium.

Definition

CP is characterized by impaired diastolic cardiac filling and elevated ventricular filling pressures due to a rigid pericardium with fusion of the visceral and parietal layers. Patients present predominantly in heart failure with elevated jugular venous pressure, dyspnea, peripheral edema, hepatomegaly and ascites.

History

Richard Lower described a patient with dyspnea and irregular pulse in 1669
Lancisi first reported a constrictive syndrome in 1828
Corrigan first described pericardial knock in 1842
Kussmaul described his sign and associated paradoxical pulse in 1873

Prevalence

Padmawati et al:	0.77 % of cardiac cases
Anand et al:	2.7 % of cardiac cases
Bawal et al:	3.0 % of cardiac cases

Age

Occurs at all age

Maximum incidence in 2nd and 3rd decade in India (Sen et al)

A decade earlier than in series from west

Gender distribution

Paul Wood:	M: F = 2:7 (female preponderance)

Female preponderance is not seen in Indian series

Sukumar et al:	Male = Female
Bashi et al:	M: F = 2.7: 1

Etiology

Inflammatory

Tuberculosis: Most common cause in Indian series

Bashi et al	61 %
Pilley et al	48 % (Autopsy series)
P L Washi	38.8 %
Sen et al	
	62.5 % (Clinical series)
	75 % (Surgically operated cases)

Viral: Especially coxsackie and echovirus

Collagen vascular disease: Rheumatoid arthritis, SLE, Scleroderma, Sarcoidosis

Following suppurative pericarditis

Post Cardiac Surgery

Trauma

Irradiation

End stage renal disease

Idiopathic: Most common cause in Western series (40 %)

Neoplasm: e.g., Breast cancer, Lung cancer, Mesothelioma, Melanoma etc.

Unusual associations

Mitral stenosis: Sen et al / Sukumar et al

Guinea worm: Sen et al (1 case)

Fungal infection

Pathology

In CP, the visceral pericardium and the parietal pericardium are fibrosed and fused together, although not necessarily always thickened. Calcification can result in the formation of pericardial calcium plaques (eggshell appearance), which may penetrate into the myocardium

CP can present as an acute or subacute case of pericarditis gradually developing constriction features or as a chronic state with no previous history of pericarditis.

Acute or subacute stage

Acute pericarditis (with effusion) gradually develops into constrictive phase within a period of 3 months to 2 years

Responsible for 30 – 45 % cases of CP

Paul Wood's series: 20% cases

Other characteristics
Affects younger patients

Female preponderance

Predominantly due to Tuberculosis

Calcification is rare

In these cases signs of cardiac compression does not disappear (if already present) after anti Koch's treatment (AKT)

Earlier the institution of AKT, lesser the chance to develop constriction (especially if started within few weeks)

Chronic phase

No history of acute pericarditis

Paul Wood: Seen in more than 75 % cases

Heavy calcification (70 % cases)

Thick, fused pericardium involving greater part of surface of both ventricles is seen in almost in all cases. Localized atrial or caval constriction is never seen.

Clinical features

Symptoms:

In decreasing order of frequency

Dyspnea on exertion

Abdominal swelling and ankle edema

Unusual fatigue

Cough

Constitutional symptoms of tuberculosis (In cases where the etiology is tuberculosis)

According to Paul Wood (based on study of 40 cases of CP), ascites and pedal edema are usually the first symptoms. Ascites is disproportionately more than the edema.

In his series these symptoms were present as follows:

Ascites with edema:	55 %
Edema alone:	15 %
Neither:	30 %
Ascites alone:	0 %

If ascites is present without pedal edema, suspect cause other than CP. The most common cause in India is tuberculous peritonitis.

In CP

1. The development of edema is more dependent on cardiac output (CO) and renal flow rather than raised venous pressure.
   The restricted distensibility of the atria, in constrictive pericarditis, limits the secretion of atrial natriuretic factor and thus, reduces its natriuretic and diuretic effects. This results in retention of water and sodium greater than that occurring in patients with edema from myocardial disease
2. For the same rise in venous pressure, CO is better maintained in CP as compared to other causes of CHF.
3. Ascites and hepatomegaly in CP are as frequent as in other cause of CHF for comparable increase in venous pressure.

Breathlessness in his series (Wood) was present in nearly all patients.

Breathlessness is due to

Decreased cardiac output (CO)

Raised diaphragm

Pleural effusion (develops sooner or later)

Increased PCWP: Pulmonary venous pressure is as high as systemic venous pressure. Pulmonary venous pressure is rarely rises high enough to cause interstitial edema and hence less likely to cause significant pulmonary hypertension. Significant pulmonary hypertension develops if pulmonary venous pressure (PVP) approaches or exceeds 25 mmHg on a chronic basis. In order to have PVP more than 25 mm Hg, the left atrial pressure (LAP) has to be more than 18 mm Hg. As there is equalization of pressure in all cardiac chambers in CP (see later in hemodynamics), the right atrial pressure (RAP) will also be near 18 mm Hg. As the signs of right sided heart failure will develop at a much lower RAP (hence low LAP) and therefore this situation (very high LAP and significant PH) is not seen in CP.

Orthopnea in CP

Wood: 46 %

Gimlette: 90 % (Series of 62 patients)

Causes:

Bilateral pleural effusion and ascites

Additional myocardial dysfunction

According to Wood, orthopnea is voluntary rather than imperative.

Signs:

1. Pulse:

Small volume

Paradoxical: In less than 50 % cases (as per Braunwald 33 %)

Pulse volume is better maintained in CP as compared to myopathic failure due to other causes (CO is better maintained in CP as compared to other causes of CHF)

2. Blood pressure:

Low-normal systolic, diastolic and pulse pressure

3. Jugular venous pulse (JVP):

Elevated in nearly 100 % cases. Normal in occult CP

A and V waves: Increased but not prominent

Sharp „y' descent: Diastolic collapse of „Friedreich'

Deep 'y' descent may be present

These waves result from high filling pressure, sudden release of pressure due to rapid tricuspid inflow, followed by a sharp rise of pressure when further expansion of ventricle is prevented by the rigid pericardium.

Positive Kussmaul's sign: Elevation of systemic venous pressures with inspiration

Inspiration causes descent of diaphragm leading to tensing of pericardium, resulting in raised JVP. Also the additional venous return of inspiration is not accommodated by RV due to rigid shield of pericardium

A common nonspecific finding in CP

Also observed in patients with

Right ventricular failure,

Restrictive cardiomyopathy,

Right ventricular infarction, and

Tricuspid stenosis

Not present in patients with cardiac tamponade

Jugular Venous Pulse in CP (Figure 1)

Feature	Findings	Mechanism / significance
Level	Elevated	Proportional to severity of CP

Waves

A wave	Never prominent	Atrial constriction does not permit exaggerated atrial contraction
X descent	Normal or exaggerated	Constriction around AV groove results in excessive descent of AV septum
V wave	Normal usually v = a	Venous return to RA is unaffected
Y descent	Rapid and steep	Rapid ventricular filling due to active ventricular relaxation encouraged by spring like pericardium. The rapid 'y' descent coincides with diastolic outward movement of the pericardium and pericardial knock

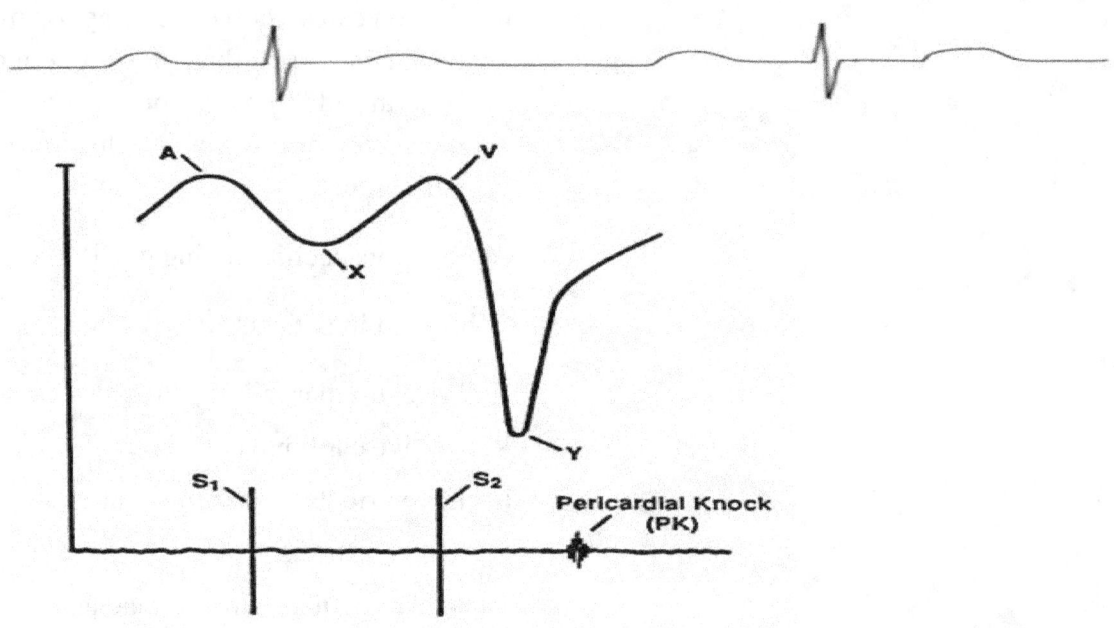

Figure 1: Jugular venous pulse waves in constrictive pericarditis, in relation to ECG and heart sounds

4. Atrial arrhythmias:
    Atrial fibrillation: 35 % cases

    Atrial flutter: 10 % cases

    > This is uncommon in Indian patients. Basir et al has reported atrial arrhythmias in 10 % of cases.

    > Presence of atrial arrhythmias is related to the duration of symptoms. Seen only in 10 % of acute CP whereas the incidence is as high as 70 % in chronic cases. Hence, presence of atrial fibrillation usually suggests chronic CP

5. Cardiac signs:
    Impalpable apex: Seen in 90 % cases

    Precordial retraction of chest due to adhesive pericarditis (Bouillard's sign)

    Heart sounds:

    > Faint

    > Precordial knock: Due to an early S 3 (A2 – S3 gap is 0.09 – 0.12 sec)

    Gallops: Both S3 and S4 may be present

6. Other signs:
    Hepatomegaly: Pulsatile hepatomegaly

    Splenomegaly

    Ascites

    Signs of protein losing enteropathy

CP: Unusual patterns

Annular CP:

Very rare

Due to constriction of pericardium in AV groove.

It behaves as functional mitral stenosis

Transverse sinus is infrequently involved in CP and hence a constriction ring around great vessels is not seen

Up to 7 % cases may have gradient between SVC and pulmonary artery

Uncommon patterns of cardiac constriction

For centuries, chronic constrictive pericarditis was the only known syndrome of cardiac constriction. More recently, other syndromes of cardiac constriction have been described, which share the characteristics of being less severe or having a shorter clinical course. These types of constrictive pericarditis frequently exhibit a hemodynamic pattern of "elastic" rather than rigid constriction, which in some way is a compressive syndrome intermediate between tamponade and rigid constriction.

Effusive–constrictive pericarditis

Effusive–constrictive pericarditis is a clinical–hemodynamic syndrome in which there is constriction of the heart by the visceral pericardium in the presence of effusion in free pericardial space.

Diagnosis:

Demonstration of persistently raised right atrial and end diastolic ventricular pressures after the intrapericardial pressure is reduced to normal levels by pericardiocentesis.

Subsequent course:

Evolves to persistent constriction requiring pericardiectomy.

Rarely, effusive–constrictive pericarditis may be transient and may resolve spontaneously, especially in idiopathic cases.

Transient cardiac constriction

Rarely a cardiac constriction could be a transient phenomenon.

Follow up cases of acute pericarditis have shown complete resolution in majority. In some cases (10-20%) recovery may be preceded by transient constriction. Some cases of acute pericarditis show evidence of subacute effusive – constrictive pericarditis and eventually develop classical CP. Some cases may directly progress to subacute or chronic constriction.

Transient constriction would represent an intermediate link between uncomplicated recovery and the severe, irreversible types of constriction.

In one study the features of constriction spontaneously resolved after a mean period of 2.7 months. Importance of this entity is that awareness of it may obviate the need for pericardiectomy.

Occult constrictive pericarditis

The term occult constrictive pericarditis was introduced in 1977 by Bush and associates. This term is used for patients, in whom physical and hemodynamic features of constriction are not apparent in their baseline state, but which are brought about by the rapid infusion of saline.

But it is a poorly standardized test and the interpretation of the findings can be quite difficult. It is better not to advise pericardiectomy solely on the basis of this test.

Patterns of cardiac constriction in different etiologies of pericardial disease

In a prospective follow up of patients with acute pericardial disease, severe subacute constriction requiring pericardiectomy developed in 56% (9/16) and 35% (6/17) of patients with tuberculous and purulent pericarditis, respectively, and in 17% (2/12) of patients with neoplastic pericarditis. In contrast, only 2 of 177 patients with acute idiopathic pericarditis developed effusive–constrictive pericarditis requiring pericardiectomy (benign transient constriction is the rule). By contrast, none of the 28 patients with massive chronic idiopathic pericardial effusion developed any feature of constriction. These patterns of constriction in the different etiologies of pericardial disease may have some clinical value for the diagnosis in individual patients

Severity of CP

1. JVP:
   Degree of elevation: Higher the elevation more severe is the CP
   Positive Kussmaul's sign suggests moderate to severe CP

2. Pericardial knock:
   Earlier the knock more severe is the CP

3. Wide split of S2 on inspiration is proportional to severity

4. Ratio of ‚x' / 'y' descent: Lower the ratio higher is the severity

5. Degree of pericardial thickening and myocardial involvement especially LV is proportional to more severe disease

6. LAE: If LA posterior wall is more than 2 cm posterior to LV posterior wall, severe CP is likely

Investigations

<u>Blood tests</u>:

Raised ESR

Liver dysfunction only in long standing cases

Pro – BNP Levels:

>Increased in pericardial diseases including CP

>Increase is due to diastolic dysfunction.

>BNP levels are even higher in restrictive cardiomyopathy and may be useful in differentiating these disorders.

<u>ECG in CP</u>

Almost always abnormal (as per Wood: abnormal in 90 % cases)

Low voltage complex: As a rule it is present.

Wide spread T wave flattening or inversion without QRS deformity

P mitrale (s/o LAE): Common

Atrial arrhythmias: 30 % cases (Western series); Not so common in India

While it is rule for these changes to persist after pericardiectomy, occasionally the ECG changes return to normal.

<u>CXR in CP</u> (Figure 2)

1. Lack of cardiomegaly
    If cardiomegaly is present, it suggests effusive constrictive pericarditis

2. Pericardial calcification:
    Wood: 50 % cases

    Freidberg: 80 % cases

    Bhargawa (India):15 % cases

3. Triangular shape of heart and loss of definition of cardiac border.

4. LAE: Bhargawa et al : 75 %

5. Relatively poor pulsation of heart border on fluoroscopy

6. Evidence of pleural effusion (Unilateral or bilateral)

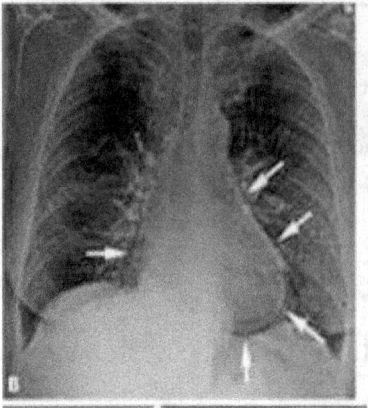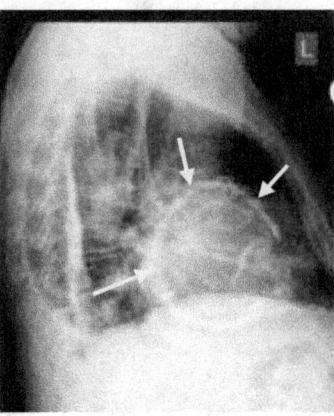

Figure 2: Chest X-ray in PA and Lateral views: It shows
pericardial calcification (arrows)

Echocardiography

*No echocardiographic finding is **pathognomonic** for constriction*

M-mode echocardiography

Diastolic "septal bounce" may be seen: In classic CP, the IVS shows a
brisk, early diastolic motion (posterior motion) toward the left
ventricle during inspiration, followed by a rebound in the opposite
direction (anterior) during expiration. This septal bounce reflects
exaggerated interventricular dependence combined with forceful
early diastolic filling.

Abrupt checking of the left ventricular posterior wall (LVPW)
diastolic movement by the rigid pericardium (coincides with the
"pericardial knock" which corresponds to the abrupt termination of
rapid ventricular filling. This lack of motion during mid diastole
and late diastole is termed "flattening," of the LV posterior wall.

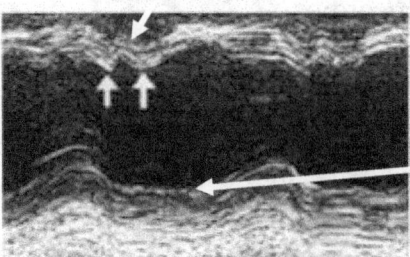

Figure 3: M mode LV showing septal bounce in IVS (short white arrows) and flattening of LVPW movement (long white arrow)

Early opening of the pulmonary valve in late diastole, due to an elevated RVEDP.

Steep E-F slope: S/O Rapid early diastolic filling

Sharp downward motion of the posterior aortic root in early diastole: Sign of rapid early diastolic filling.

Thickened pericardium

Differentiation between CP and RCMP can be assisted by Digitization of M mode echocardiograms

The following variables are measured:

(a) Left ventricular cavity size is measured both at end diastole (EDD (cm)) and end systole (ESD (cm)) (taken as those dimensions synchronous with the Q wave of the electrocardiogram and A2 on the phonocardiogram respectively).

(b) Fractional shortening (FS (%)) is derived: FS = (EDD - ESD) / EDD.

(c) Peak rate of increase of left ventricular dimension during early diastole (LV max rate (cm/s) (this represents peak left ventricular filling rate).

(d) Peak rate of reduction of left ventricle dimension during systole (LV min rate (cm/s)) (this represents peak left ventricular emptying rate).

(e) Posterior wall thickness at minimum cavity size (PW min (cm)).

(f) Posterior wall thickness at maximum cavity size (PW max (cm)) and

(g) Percentage systolic thickening of posterior wall (%PW) derived from: (PW min- PW max) / PW min x 100.

(h) Peak rate of thinning of posterior wall during early diastole (PW max rate (cm/s)).

(X) Peak rate of thickening of posterior wall during systole (PW min rate (cm/s)).

(j) Septal thickness at minimum cavity size (sept min (cm))

RCMP: Significantly lower values than controls

FS
LV max rate
LV min rate
% PW
PW max rate
PW min rate
Slower ventricular filling and emptying (with an associated reduced amplitude of wall motion and rate of posterior wall thinning and thickening) than the controls.
% PW, PW max rate and PW min rate are significantly lower than values in CP

For diagnostic purposes peak rate of thinning of the posterior wall during early diastole is the best discriminant.

2 D Features

Septal bounce: Most consistent finding in 2 D echo in CP

Angle between the posterior LV wall and posterior left atrium: In CP it can be blunted, because the thickened, constricting pericardium affects the posterior left ventricle more than the posterior left atrium, which then expands at a more acute angle respective to the LV wall.

Abnormal left atrial-left ventricular junction with an angle between posterior walls of the left atrium and ventricle less than 150° is indicative of CP

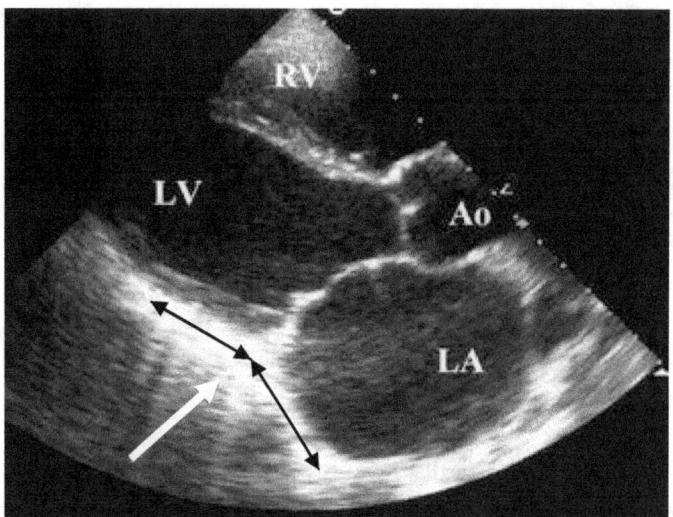

Figure4: PLAX view shows an angle (thick white arrow) between posterior wall of LV and LA (Black arrows).An angle < 150 favors constrictive pericarditis.

Left atrial enlargement and RA enlargement

Normal size and systolic function of ventricles

Thickened pericardium: *TEE is more sensitive in detecting pericardial thickness*

Color Doppler

Mild mitral and tricuspid regurgitation
>Severe mitral and tricuspid regurgitation is not seen in isolated or predominant constrictive physiology and are markers for underlying myocardial disease

Mitral inflow as assessed by Doppler echocardiography demonstrates an increased early diastolic filling velocity followed by rapid deceleration, leading to a short filling period. Early mitral inflow deceleration time is usually, but not always, 160 ms. In CP, early diastolic mitral inflow is reduced with the onset of inspiration, and isovolumic relaxation time is prolonged. With expiration, mitral inflow returns to normal, and isovolumic relaxation time shortens. Typically, patients with CP demonstrate an increase in early diastolic mitral inflow velocity of 25% during expiration compared with inspiration.

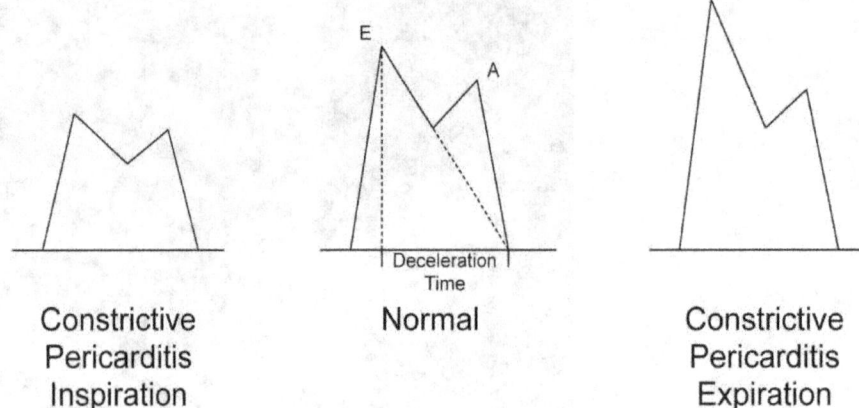

Constrictive   Normal   Constrictive
Pericarditis   Pericarditis
Inspiration   Expiration

Figure5: Inflow across mitral valve

RV and LV inflow show prominent E wave due to rapid early
    diastolic filling
Short deceleration time (DT) for E wave as filling abruptly
    stops due to constriction.DT < 160 ms (Normal 160-240
    ms)
Small A wave as little filling occurs during atrial contraction
E / A ratio: > 1.5:1 (Normal 0.9 – 1.5)
IVRT (Isovolumic relaxation time; time between aortic valve
    closure to mitral valve opening) < 60 ms (Normal 70-90
    ms)

Respiratory variation in MV inflow velocity (> 25%; Expiration >
    Inspiration) and in TV inflow velocity (>40%; Inspiration >
    Expiration): Due to dissociation of intrathoracic pressure from
    intracardiac pressure and enhanced ventricular interdependence

The respiratory variations are usually greater in constriction than
    in restriction (probably because of the normal
    interventricular septum), usually with greater than 25%
    changes at the onset of inspiration and expiration. Reflecting
    this, the deceleration time of the mitral Doppler inflow E
    wave is usually less than 150 ms with constriction, with a
    further decrease with inspiration. If a concomitant pericardial
    effusion is present, it may account for some respiratory
    variation.

The transtricuspid velocities show an opposite pattern to the
    transmitral (i.e., increasing with inspiration and decreasing
    with expiration). More than 40 % variation in TV inflow

velocities is suggestive of CP. The shortened deceleration time from these peak velocities is felt to correspond to the dip-and-plateau hemodynamics seen with limited early diastolic flow. The pulmonary vein Doppler inflow pattern also has respiratory variation, with its diastolic inflow being greater than systolic inflow, which itself may even reverse

Patients with RCMP and up to 20% of patients with CP may lack the typical respiratory changes in the presence of mixed constrictive-restrictive disease and/or markedly increased left atrial pressure.

Measurements of diastolic function are load-dependent (i.e., dependent on preload and afterload). If atrial and ventricular filling pressures are low, Doppler interrogation findings may be falsely negative. Likewise, if atrial and ventricular filling pressures are high, respiratory variation may be masked. *In such cases, preload may be reduced with either medication or dynamic maneuvers, such as tilting the patient's head up or having the patient sit. These maneuvers may unmask respiratory variation*

Atrial fibrillation complicates the interpretation of respiratory variation of Doppler velocities, but respiratory variation can still be appreciated **regardless of cardiac cycle length**. Usually, this requires longer recording periods of Doppler tracings.

PASP < 55 mm Hg: Severe PH excludes CP (see page 8 / symptoms for explanation)

Hepatic vein flow: Show marked diastolic flow reversal, which increases in expiration compared with inspiration.

Hepatic vein expiratory diastolic reversal ratio ≥ 0.79 (Hepatic vein diastolic reversal velocity / diastolic forward flow velocity) is an independent variable associated with CP

Compare from RCMP where diastolic hepatic vein flow reversal is more prominent with inspiration

Pulmonary vein flow: Marked respiratory variation.
The pulmonary venous systolic wave and early diastolic wave velocities, especially the early diastolic wave velocity, are increased during expiration and decreased during inspiration. (More pronounced than MV inflow).
In contrast, patients with RCMP show blunting of the systolic wave velocity and a decrease in the ratio of systolic to early diastolic wave velocity throughout the respiratory cycle,

with a large atrial reversal wave and without any significant respiratory variation.

D/D of phasic respiratory changes in mitral inflow
1. CP
2. Chronic obstructive pulmonary disease
3. Severe RV dysfunction and
4. Large respiratory variations in intrathoracic pressure

In such patients, a marked increase in inspiratory superior vena cava systolic forward flow can be helpful to rule out CP.

Color Doppler tissue imaging (DTI)

Epicardial motion was found to be reduced, approaching that of the pericardium, whereas the endocardium was moving more vigorously

Actual endocardial and epicardial tissue velocities are measured. Because myocardial relaxation itself is preserved in pure constrictive pericarditis, the early relaxation myocardial velocity (Em, also known as Ea) is normal, whereas it is abnormal with restriction (when intrinsic myocardial disease is present). For example, given that a normal Em is more than 10 cm/s, a near-normal (>8 cm/s) Em supports constriction, whereas a much lower Em supports restriction.

Longitudinal mitral annular motion by pulsed tissue Doppler and color DTI: it estimates LV relaxation

    In CP, mechanoelastic properties of the myocardium are relatively preserved in the longitudinal direction and therefore longitudinal deformation of the LV base and longitudinal early diastolic velocities are either normal or exaggerated.

    In contrast, patients with RCMP and intrinsic myocardial abnormalities have reduced longitudinal deformation of the LV base and reduced early diastolic longitudinal velocities.

A lateral or septal early diastolic mitral annular velocity of 8 cm/s on pulsed tissue Doppler is the accepted cutoff value to distinguish patients with CP from those with RCMP. Lateral e' less than septal e' (**Annulus reversus**) is more definitive of CP. Mitral annular velocities are particularly useful in CP when pronounced respiratory variations in peak early mitral in flow velocities are not seen.

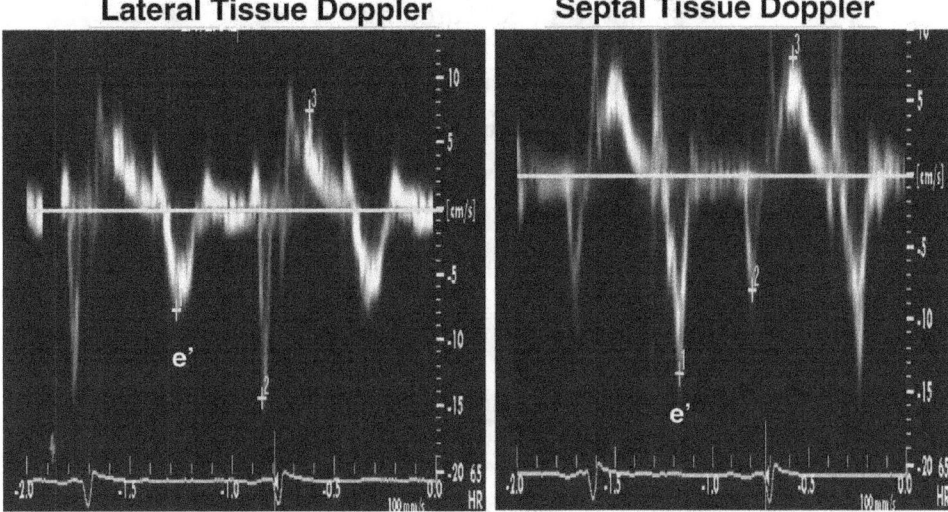

Figure 6: e' velocity > 8 cm/sec favors constrictive pericarditis over restrictive cardiomyopathy. Lateral e' less than septal e' (Annulus reverses) is characteristic of CP.

To summarize, Tissue Doppler measures myocardial tissue velocity and provides a non-invasive evaluation of myocardial relaxation. The early diastolic mitral annular velocity (e') which reflects the status of LV myocardial relaxation is reduced in most forms of heart failure related to myocardial disease, including restrictive cardiomyopathy. The normal e' velocity from the medial mitral annulus is 10 cm/sec or greater, and it is usually 6cm/sec or less in patients with a myopathy. In contrast, e' is usually preserved or even increased in constrictive pericarditis since the lateral motion of the heart is limited by the constrictive pericardium. Furthermore, the medial mitral annular e' velocity is usually greater than the lateral mitral annular e'. This again stands in contrast to what is expected in other forms of heart failure, and may reflect tethering of the lateral annulus by the constrictive process

From a Doppler perspective:

Constriction

Myocardium and myocardial compliance are normal:

Permits rapid early diastolic filling

Enhances ventricular interaction

Ventricular pressure interdependence

23

Restraint from pericardium

Abrupt termination of diastolic filling by the limit imposed by the constricting pericardium.

Restriction

Myocardium is abnormal with reduced compliance

No restraint from pericardium

Therefore, both physiologies have abnormal early diastolic filling with early atrial ventricular pressure equilibration.

<u>Ventricular pressure interdependence</u>:

In simple words, filling of one ventricle significantly impacts the filling of other ventricle.

With inspiration, the right ventricular inflow is increased, which is believed to cause the interventricular septum to shift toward the left, thus further diminishing left ventricular filling. As a result of this preload mismatch, stroke volume is augmented in the right ventricle and reduced in the left ventricle. These ventricular pressure responses have been termed discordant.

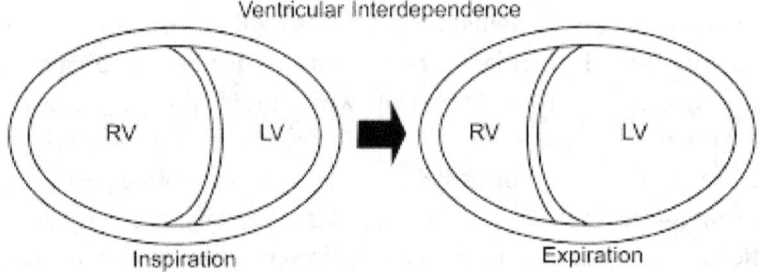

Figure 7: A simple diagram to explain ventricular interdependence

Due to this ventricular pressure interdependence, the echo-Doppler or the hemodynamic tracings obtained simultaneously in both ventricles show that the left ventricular pressure falls with inspiration while the right ventricular pressure rises. The opposite is true during expiration. This phenomenon does not occur in congestive heart failure or restrictive disorders.

Intrathoracic/intracardiac pressure disassociation

Normally intrathoracic and intracardiac pressures are related.

Inspiration reduces intrathoracic pressure which usually is fully transmitted to intracardiac pressures, but in constriction, the intracardiac pressures falls much less than intrathoracic pressure because of pericardial constraint. This difference in pressure change with inspiration results in reduced filling to left side of the heart (decrease in pressure gradient for filling the LV). The reduction in left heart filling during inspiration causes a reduction in mitral inflow velocity and a shift of the interventricular septum toward the left ventricle. With expiration, left heart filling increases which shifts the interventricular septum back toward the right ventricle, leading to reduced filling to right side of the heart and a late-diastolic reversal of flow in the hepatic veins. This intrathoracic / intracardiac dissociation occurs commonly although not exclusively) in constrictive pericarditis. This dissociation does occur, although to a much lesser extent, in restrictive cardiomyopathy.

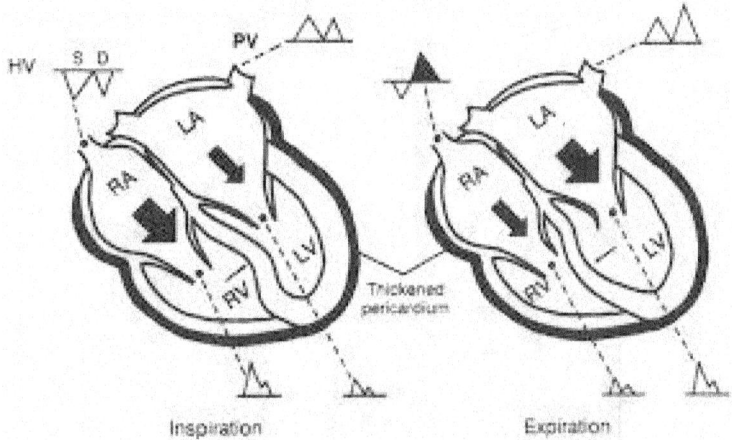

Inspiration   Expiration

Figure 8: Explains echocardiographic findings in constrictive pericarditis due to ventricular interdependence and intracardiac pressure dissociation. For details refer to "Oh JK, Hatle L, Seward JB, et al. (1994) Diagnostic role of Doppler echocardiography in constrictive pericarditis. J Am Coll Cardiol 23:154–162"

The patient's diastolic filling pressures can affect hemodynamic measurements, and some authors advocate infusing isotonic sodium chloride solution if the patient's left ventricular end-diastolic pressure is less than 15 mm Hg to unmask occult constrictive pericarditis

Summary of echocardiographic findings to differentiate CP with Restrictive CMP:

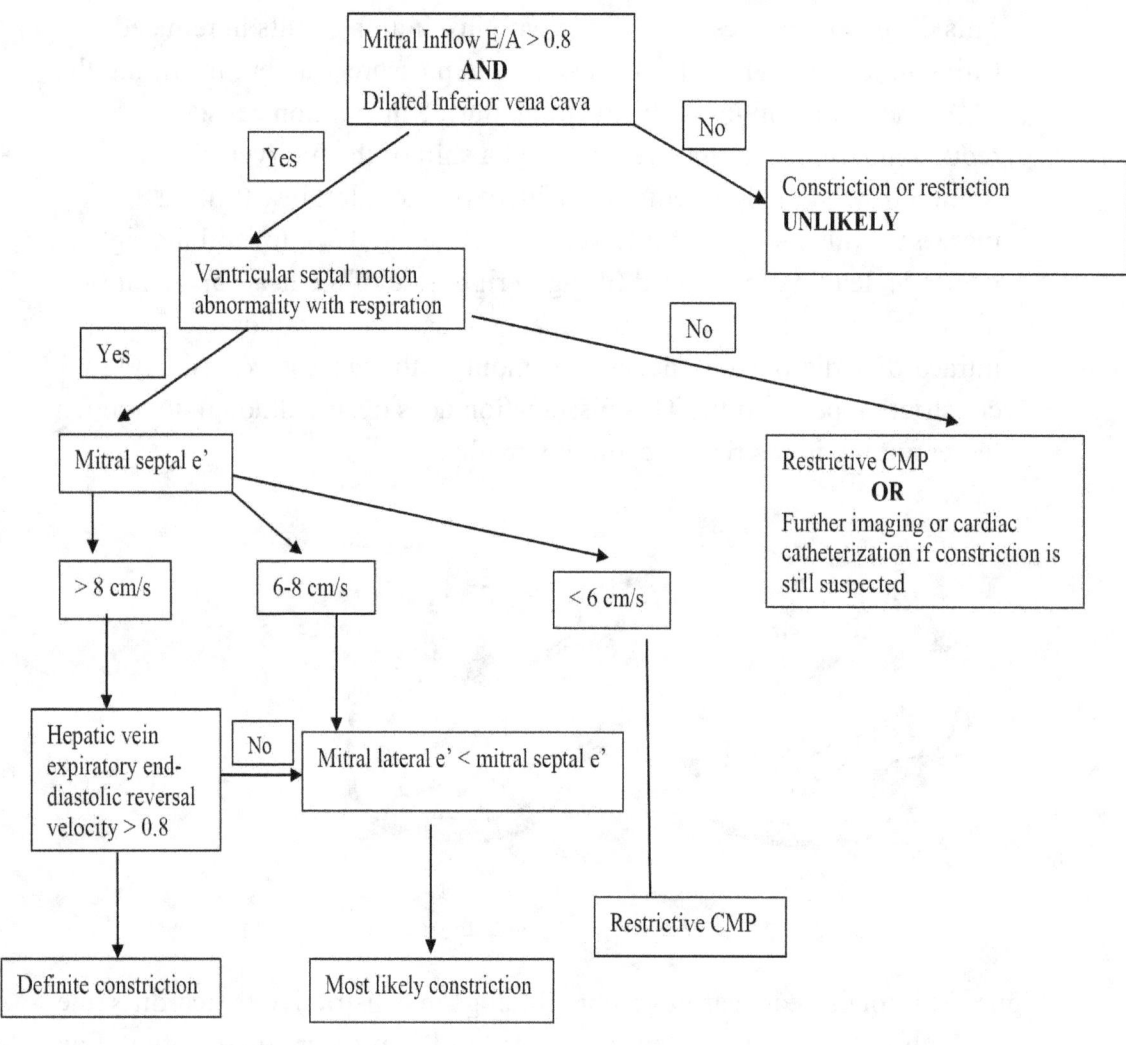

The echocardiographic findings in patients with tuberculous pericarditis

Small/moderate/large amount of pericardial effusion

Cardiac tamponade

Fibrin strand/mass-like exudate

Thickened pericardium

Constrictive pericarditis

Angiography:

Gold standard for diagnosis of CP

Hemodynamic criteria used in the diagnosis of CP are neither sensitive nor specific and they significantly overlap with those of restrictive diseases that can also alter the diastolic filling properties.

The criteria are the following:

Equalization of End-diastolic pressures: The difference between the left and the right ventricular end-diastolic pressures is 5 mm Hg or less.

Pulmonary artery pressure is less than 55 mm Hg.

The right ventricular end-diastolic pressure divided by the right ventricular end- systolic pressure is greater than 1/3.

A dip-and-plateau diastolic pressure morphology, as reflected by height of the left ventricular rapid filling wave (>7 mm Hg) is present.

The Kussmaul's sign is present: The mean right atrial pressure does not decrease during inspiration.

Ultimately, the diagnosis must be confirmed surgically at the time of complete pericardiectomy.

Hemodynamic findings:

Characteristic hemodynamic changes in CP are attributed to isolation of the cardiac chambers from intrathoracic respiratory pressure changes and a fixed end-diastolic ventricular volume

Atrial pressure:

Raised LAP and RAP

LAP (m) > RAP (m)

Difference is less than 6 mm Hg (Wood)

Wave pattern: W or M pattern

Sharp „y' descent

Deep 'y' trough

Sharp „x' descent

Increased „a' wave but not giant „a'; with well marked „v' wave; usually v is more than a; a is more than v in cardiomyopathy

Severity of CP based on wave forms

Ratio of depth of 'x' descent and depth of 'y' descent

High ratio i.e., increased depth of 'x' descent indicates less severe disease.

Ventricular pressure:

Square root response: Rapid early dip followed by a sharp rise of diastolic pressure to a high plateau which is maintained during greater part of diastole

In constrictive pericarditis, early ventricular filling during the first third of diastole is unimpeded, but, afterwards, the stiff pericardium affects flow and hemodynamics. That is, ventricular pressure decreases rapidly early and then increases abruptly to a level that is sustained until systole.

There is only a small „a' wave rise of diastolic pressure. Early 'dip' may reach at or near baseline

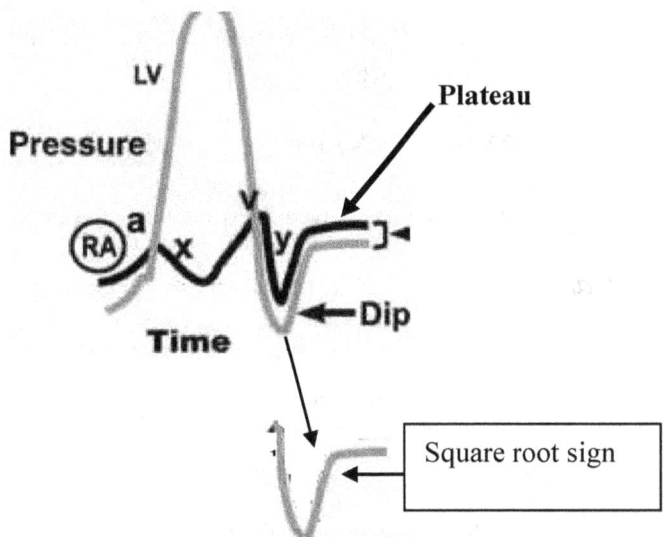

Figure 9: LV pressure in diastole showing square root response.

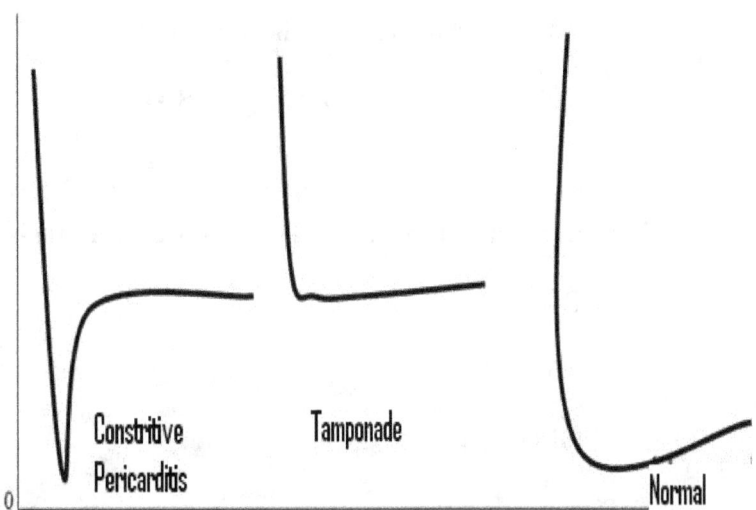

Figure 10: Note the patterns in LV diastolic pressure in constrictive pericarditis (dip and plateau), in tamponade (high and plateau due to pandiastolic resistance to ventricular filling) and in normal individuals.

Raised EDP

Both LVEDP and RVEDP are high and equal. The difference between the two is less than 5 mm Hg

Equalization of RAP (m), LAP (m), RVEDP and LVEDP is the hallmark of CP

All cardiac diastolic pressures become nearly equal. This limits end-diastolic volume, which, in turn, decreases stroke volume and cardiac output.

RVEDP / RVSP (Peak) is more than 1/3

Valsalva maneuver: Square wave response

Cardiac output (CO) and AV O2 difference

Increased CO and low AV O2 difference as compared to cardiomyopathy

Pulmonary artery pressure:

Mildly increase in PASP (PASP is almost never more than 50 mm Hg) in CP

Normal PAP (m)

High PADP (Due to high mean LAP)

PAWP = PADP = RVEDP = RAP (m)

Dip-and-plateau pattern: Differential diagnosis

CP

RCMP

COPD

Differential diagnosis of diastolic pressure equalization include

Constrictive pericarditis,

Restrictive cardiomyopathy,

Cardiac tamponade,

COPD and pneumothorax (pulmonary hyperinflation),

Dilated cardiomyopathy (if severe, all filling pressures are high),

Atrial septal defect and volume depletion (all filling pressures are low).

CT or MRI scan

The normal pericardium is 1 mm thick on CT scans or MRI scans; thickening greater than 3 mm is abnormal.

Pericardial thickening of more than 4 mm assists in differentiating constrictive disease from restrictive cardiomyopathy and a thickening of more than 6 mm adds even more specificity for constriction.

False-negative results may occur if a long-standing thin pericardial scar without appreciable thickening is present. *That is, normal pericardial thickness does not exclude pericardial constriction.*

If the hemodynamics and presentation are otherwise compatible, the diagnosis must still be entertained despite unremarkable pericardial imaging.

Both CT and MRI of the heart can identify pericardial thickening much better than echocardiography, and are probably the **most sensitive imaging techniques** currently available for delineating the morphology and thickness of the pericardium.

Ventricular function in CP

Determining the relative contribution of pericardial restraint versus myocardial dysfunction in such patients remains a diagnostic challenge.

Co existing ventricular dysfunction is present in CP if following criteria are seen:

1. Delayed early dip and slow rise to raised diastolic pressure in RV pressure trace is suggestive of coexisting myocardial involvement (Sukumar et al)
2. Failure of cardiac index to increase with exercise
3. Histamine infusion (Cindell et al):Histamine infusion increases cardiac output if there is preexisting myocardial dysfunction
4. Insignificant increase in cardiac output with acute digitalization (Grover et al)
5. Fall of cardiac index at high rate of right atrial pacing (Bhatia et al)

Insignificant increase in hemodynamic response to acute digitalization was the only parameter which clearly distinguished patients with poor myocardial function

Inadequate relief of symptoms after pericardiectomy is due to

(Bhatia et al)

Inadequate surgical decortication

Associated myocardial dysfunction

Delayed resolution due to unknown factors

Treatment

1. Medical treatment

Medical therapy should never delay surgery

Useful in

1. Therapy of specific etiologies (i.e. tuberculous pericarditis)

   May prevent the progression to constriction.

   Antituberculosis antibiotics may significantly reduce the risk of constriction from >80% to <10%

2. Therapy (generally based on anti-inflammatory drugs) may solve the transient constriction

   The detection of elevated CRP and imaging evidence of pericardial inflammation by contrast enhancement on CT and/or MRI may be helpful to identify patients with potentially reversible forms of constriction where empiric anti-inflammatory therapy should be considered and may prevent the need for pericardiectomy.

3. Therapy is supportive and aimed at controlling symptoms of congestion in advanced cases and when surgery is contraindicated or is at high risk.

Treatment options

Anti Koch's treatment (AKT): When the etiology is tuberculosis

As per ESC guidelines

Tuberculostatic treatment combined with steroids might be associated with fewer deaths, less frequent need for pericardiocentesis or pericardiectomy (level of evidence A, indication IIb).

If given, prednisone should be administered in relatively high doses (1–2 mg/kg per day) since rifampicin induces its liver metabolism. This dosage is maintained for 5–7 days and is progressively reduced to discontinuation in 6–8 weeks.

Anti failure treatment: Routine antifailure treatment

Digoxin should be given post pericardiectomy if symptoms persist. Additional myocardial dysfunction is usual cause in such cases.

2. Surgical treatment

Pericardiectomy: It should be as complete as possible

Complete pericardiectomy is the definitive therapy and is a potential cure.

Performed through left thoracolateral incision

Other common cardiac surgeries performed through left thoracolateral technique are;

PDA ligation
Closed Mitral valvotomy
Diseases of aortic arch and descending thoracic aorta (eg.,Coarctation)
BT shunt

Pericardiectomy relieves pericardial restraint and in the absence of concomitant myocardial dysfunction, effectively restores diastolic filling.

Pericardiectomy is the accepted standard of treatment in patients with chronic constrictive pericarditis who have persistent and prominent symptoms. However, surgery should be considered cautiously in patients with either mild or very advanced disease and in those with radiation-induced constriction, myocardial dysfunction or significant renal dysfunction

Patients with „end-stage' constrictive pericarditis derive little or no benefit from pericardiectomy, and the operative risk is inordinately high.

Results are generally better if the procedure is performed earlier in the course, when less calcification is present and when the chance of abnormal myocardium or advanced heart failure is reduced.

Some judgment is required because patients who are asymptomatic (NYHA class I) or who have early NYHA stage II symptoms may be clinically stable for years.

Pericardial decortication should be as extensive as possible, especially at the diaphragmatic-ventricular contact regions.

After complete pericardiectomy mitral inflow patterns return to normal, and little respiratory variation is seen on Doppler echocardiography. Accordingly, Doppler assessment of respiratory variation has been reported to be useful for evaluating the outcome of pericardiectomy.

Patients who had minimal respiratory variation after pericardiectomy were asymptomatic compared with those who continued to show respiratory variation.

Poor surgical results are observed in patients with organ failure (especially renal and hepatic), ascites, uncorrected coronary artery disease, myocardial fibrosis, older age, NYHA class IV, or postradiation pericarditis.

Prior ionizing radiation is associated with a poor long-term outcome, because it induces cardiomyopathy as well as pericardial disease

The published surgical mortality rates range from 5-15%. Significantly, 80-90% of patients who undergo pericardiectomy, postoperatively achieve NYHA class I or II.

Only 50% of patients respond to surgery, but in many patients, the symptoms dramatically resolve

Mortality: 5-15 %

Results

Excellent:	52 %
Good:	30 %
Poor:	7 %

AKT should be continued for 1 yr after surgery

Prognosis

Long-term survival after pericardiectomy depends on the underlying cause.

	Survival at 7 yrs
Idiopathic CP	88% (best prognosis)

Post cardiac surgery	66%
Postradiation CP	27% (worst prognosis)

Even after adequate pericardiectomy:

Venous pressure may remain high

Kussmaul's sign may remain positive

S3 is present; although it is softer and delayed

ECG: Usually unchanged

Normal rhythm is seldom restored if atrial arrhythmias were present preoperatively

CXR features also may not show much difference

Reconstriction is not observed post pericardiectomy

D/D between Active CP (Effusive-constrictive) and Chronic CP

Findings	ACP (%)	CCP (%)
Paradoxical pulse	50	15
JVP		
Dominant x descent	75	17
Dominant y descent	25	58
AF / A Flutter	10	70
LV apical impulse		Less common (10 %)
MR / TR	Rare	Rare
S3	same	same
ECG		
Normal	10	16
T wave abnormality	90	84
CXR		
Calcification	-	70
Cardiomegaly	60 (effusive)	0
Pleural effusion	90	Rare
Catheterization data	similar	similar

Differential diagnosis with Restrictive Cardiomyopathy

Features	CP	RCMP
Paradoxical pulse	33 %	Rare
Blood pressure		
	Normal	Variable (Postural hypotension in amyloidosis)
Pulse pressure	Well preserved	
JVP		
Giant 'a'	Rare	Present (42 %)
„a' and 'v'	Small and equal	a > v
		If TR then v > a
X descent	Preserved	Absent with
		TR and RVF
Y	Deep and rapid	May be present
Kussmaul's sign	Present	Variable (+/-)
A. Fibrillation	50 % (India 10%)	33 %
Apex beat	Impalpable or systolic retraction	LV type
Pulsation in LICS (3rd ICS)	Diastolic	Systolic (seen not felt; due to dilated RVOT)
Pulsation in LICS (2nd ICS)	Absent	Present (s/o PH)
Hepatic pulsation	Diastolic	Systolic
Cardiomegaly	Absent (Present with effusive CP)	Present
Pericardial knock	50 %	Absent
S3/S4 gallop	Absent	Variable (+/-)
MR / TR	Rare; less than mild	Common

ECG

Normal	15 %	10 %
BBB	Absent	25 %
LVH	Absent	30 %
Q – T pattern	Absent	+/-
T inversion (V1-V6)	80 – 90 %	30 %

CXR

Cardiomegaly	+/-	++ (85 %)
	+ s/o effusive CP	
Pericardial Calcification	70 % (India 15 %)	Absent
Pleural effusion	++ (Effusive CP)	Rare
Pericardial thickening	++	Normal
	> 4 mm on CT / MRI	
	> 8 mm on Cath	

Hemodynamics

LAP (m) – RAP (m)	0-6 mm Hg	10 – 20 mm Hg
PASP / RVSP	Normal/mildly high	High> 45 mm Hg with LVEMF
RVEDP - LVEDP	0 – 5 mm Hg	> 5 mm Hg
RVSP / RVEDP	< 3	> 3
PEP / LVET	0.31	0.48 (s/o systolic dysfunction)
CO	4 – 5 L/min	About 3.5 L/min
< 2.5 L/min	25 %	80 %
A-V O2 Difference	≈ 50 ml/L	≈ 75 ml/L
> 55 ml/L	30 %	90 %

LV filling

(Early diastole)	> 80 %	< 50 %
Crista Supraventricular motion		
	Normal	Global decrease
	(Even with RV dysfunction)	
Coronary Arteries	Displaced	Normal
	(From epicardium)	
Endomyocardial biopsy	Normal	Myopathic findings (60 -70 %)
Pericardial biopsy	Diagnostic	

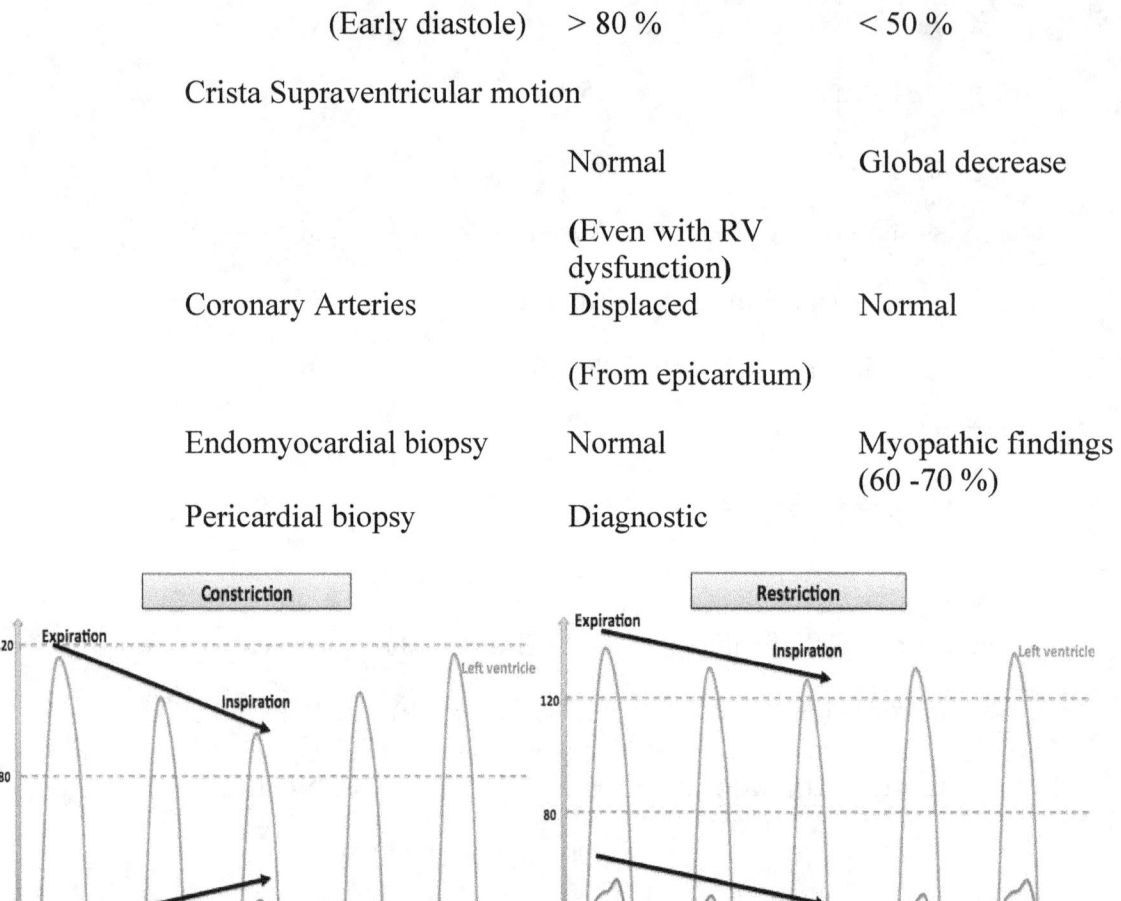

Figure 11: Ventricular interdependence and intracardiac pressure dissociation in constrictive pericarditis cause decrease in LV peak pressure and increase in RV peak pressure during inspiration. However in restrictive cardiomyopathy both pressures decrease with inspiration.

Kussmaul criteria for prediction of CP:

LVEDP – RVEDP (< 5 mm Hg):

      CP: 92 %
      CMP: 70 %
      Predictive value: 85 %
RVSP ≤ 50 mm Hg:

      CP: 90 %
      CMP: 24 %
      Predictive value: 70 %
RVEDP/ RVSP (≥ 0.33):

CP: 95 %
CMP: 32 %
Predictive value: 76 %
If all criteria are present the predictive value is more than 90 %

Indian Series

Bashi, ..., John S et al

N = 118

Symptom class

NYHA Class $\geq$ 3:	97 (82 %)

Ascites or edema: 100 (85 %)

Raised JVP: 100 %

Hepatomegaly: 100 %

Muffled Heart sounds: 98 %

Cardiomegaly: 50 %

Etiology

Tuberculosis: 72 (61 %)

Hospital mortality: 11 %

Follow Up: 72

NYHA Class $\leq$ 2: 63

Endomyocardial Fibrosis

(Idiopathic Restrictive Cardiomyopathy)

Restrictive Cardiomyopathy (RCMP)

Cardiomyopathy: Classification

Hypertrophic cardiomyopathy

Dilated cardiomyopathy

Restrictive cardiomyopathy

Arrhythmogenic right ventricular cardiomyopathy

Unclassified cardiomyopathy
> Left ventricular noncompaction
> Takotsubo cardiomyopathy

Restrictive cardiomyopathy (RCMP) is a rare disease of the myocardium and is less common as compared to hypertrophic or dilated cardiomyopathies. Its principal abnormality is diastolic dysfunction; specifically, restricted ventricular filling. RCMP accounts for approximately 5% of all cases of primary heart muscle disease.

The World Health Organization (WHO) defines RCMP as a myocardial disease characterized by restrictive filling and reduced diastolic volume of either or both ventricles with normal or near-normal systolic function and wall thickness. Increased interstitial fibrosis may be present. This disease may be idiopathic or associated with other diseases. The course of RCMP varies, depending on the pathology and treatment, but is often unsatisfactory.

The importance of an accurate diagnosis of RCMP is to distinguish this condition from <u>constrictive pericarditis,</u> a clinically and hemodynamically similar entity that also presents with restrictive physiology but is frequently curable by surgical intervention. This distinction is difficult to make but crucial because the treatment options and prognoses for the 2 conditions differ drastically.

Causes of RCMP

Idiopathic

Infiltrative and storage disease

<u>Hemochromatosis</u>

<u>Amyloidosis</u> (the most common cause of RCMP in the United States)

<u>Sarcoidosis</u>

Carcinoid heart disease

Glycogen storage disease of the heart

Progressive systemic sclerosis (scleroderma)

Familial cardiomyopathy

Anthracycline toxicity and other drugs such as Methysergide, Busulfan, Serotonin, Ergotamine etc.

Radiation

Malignancy

Endomyocardial Fibrosis

Definition

Endomyocardial fibrosis (EMF) is an idiopathic disorder of the tropical and subtropical regions of the world that is characterized by the development of restrictive cardiomyopathy

History

Arthur Williams (1938): Described „patches of fibrosis in the ventricles' of 2 Ugandan patients

J N P Davies (1955): Detailed description of pathological features and labeled the dense fibrous plaques of mural endocardium as "endomyocardial fibrosis"

Brockington and Olsen (1979): Proposed role of eosinophils in causation of EMF due to similarity to Loffler's EMF

Synonyms

Davies' Disease

EMF (Endomyocardial fibrosis)

Fibroelastic Endocarditis

Loeffler Endomyocardial Fibrosis with Eosinophilia

Loeffler Fibroplastic Parietal Endocarditis

Loeffler's Disease

Epidemiology

India: This disease occurs only in certain pockets of the world. The disease is most common in the tropics 15° on either side of the equator. Kerala was considered as the hot spot for the disease with isolated reports from rest of India. In Kerala during late 1970s and 1980s, 2.5 per cent of all cardiac admissions below the age of 40 years were contributed by patients with EMF

The disease continues as the commonest cause of restrictive cardiomyopathy in Africa where it is a public health problem.

More than half of all EMF cases are diagnosed during the first decade of life and a second peak incidence occurs in women of childbearing age

(Bimodal peak). Adult preponderance has been found in young women from Uganda, but in Mozambique, males were more commonly affected, while in other studies, both sexes were equally affected

Pathology

In EMF, the underlying process produces patchy fibrosis of the endocardial surface of the heart, leading to reduced compliance and, ultimately, restrictive physiology as the endomyocardial surface becomes more generally involved. Endocardial fibrosis principally involves the apices of the right and left ventricles and may affect the atrioventricular valves mainly by tethering the papillary muscles, leading to tricuspid and mitral regurgitation.

Olsen described 3 phases of EMF.

First phase:

Eosinophilic infiltration of the myocardium with necrosis of the subendocardium. Pathological picture is consistent with acute myocarditis.

Seen in the first 5 weeks of the illness.

Second stage:

Typically observed after 10 months,

Is associated with thrombus formation over the initial lesions, with a decrement in the amount of inflammatory activity.

Third phase:

Fibrotic phase

Seen after several years of disease activity.

Endocardium is replaced by collagenous fibrosis. Extensive calcification is rarely associated with fibrosis. *This pathomorphologic schema is not observed uniformly and has not been consistently supported by other investigators.*

The basic feature of the disease is the formation of fibrous tissue on the endocardium of the inflow tract of the right or left ventricle or both, and to a lesser extent in the myocardium. Endomyocardial fibrosis may become so prominent that it leads to partial obliteration of one or both ventricles with decreased ventricular distensibility and impaired diastolic filling. The fibrotic process is usually located at the apex of the affected ventricle and extends to the inflow tract. Involvement of the chordae tendinae is frequent and causes mitral and/or tricuspid regurgitation.

Etiopathogenesis

Unclear: A specific single etiology of EMF has not been established.

EMF is most frequently observed in the socially disadvantaged and in children and young women.

Suggested potential causes include the following:

Infectious causes

Parasites (e.g., helminths)

Protozoans (e.g., toxoplasmosis, malaria)

Inflammatory causes - Eosinophilia

Nutritional causes

General malnutrition

High-tuber diet

Cerium toxicity

Hypomagnesemia

In regions of sub-Saharan Africa where the disease is most prevalent, the typical diet is high in a tuber called cassava, which contains relatively high concentrations of the rare earth element cerium (Ce). The combination of high Ce levels and hypomagnesemia has been shown to produce EMF-like lesions in laboratory animals.

Severe prolonged eosinophilia from any cause (e.g., allergic, autoimmune, parasitic, leukemic, or idiopathic) can lead to eosinophilic infiltration of the myocardium. The intracytoplasmic granular content of activated eosinophils is believed to be responsible for the toxic damage to the heart. This eosinophilic cardiomyopathy, also known as Loeffler endocarditis, is associated with dense EMF, intraventricular thrombus formation, and obliteration of the ventricular cavity in its late stages; accordingly, it is included in the category of obliterative RCMP.

EMF, which is observed exclusively in equatorial Africa and less frequently in Asia and South America, was believed to be the end stage of eosinophilic endomyocarditis. However, **it now is considered a separate entity because it does not exhibit eosinophilia.** EMF demonstrates pathology that is similar to that described above (Loeffler endocarditis) and therefore is grouped under obliterative RCMP.

Tropical EMF and Löeffler endocarditis should be distinguished from endocardial fibroelastosis, which is characterized by cartilaginous thickening of the mural endocardium, chiefly of the left ventricle. This disease is most common in the first 2 years of life and in some patients, appears to be an inherited disorder that is associated with congenital cardiac malformations.

Clinical Features

Symptoms

Typically, endomyocardial fibrosis (EMF) has an insidious onset, and symptoms relate to the specific chambers and valves where the disease is most extensive.

When right ventricular involvement or tricuspid regurgitation predominates, lower extremity swelling, increasing abdominal girth and nausea may be expected. Rarely cyanosis and clubbing are present.

With left ventricular involvement, dyspnea is the predominant symptom, especially exertional dyspnea. Additionally, fatigue, paroxysmal nocturnal dyspnea and orthopnea may be present.

Symptoms worsens due to AF development

Physical Examination:

Physical findings are also dependent on the extent and distribution of disease.

In those with right ventricular involvement, jugular venous pressure elevation, ascites and edema may be present. The presence of ascites may appear out of proportion to the amount of peripheral edema. This may occur because of the concomitant presence of a protein-losing enteropathy and subsequent hypoalbuminemia.

Patients with tricuspid regurgitation may have giant V waves observed in the jugular venous pulsations.

A third or fourth heart sound and tachycardia may be present.

Signs of pulmonary congestion are present in patients with left-sided disease

To summarize, the triad of elevated jugular venous pressure, ascites and hepatomegaly form the hallmark of right ventricular EMF, which can present with cyanosis and clubbing because of stretch opening of foramen ovale. Mild cardiomegaly, loud left ventricular third heart sound, short systolic murmur and severe pulmonary hypertension form the hallmark for the diagnosis of left ventricular endomyocardial fibrosis

Investigations

CXR:

Characteristic feature

Cardiomegaly is secondary to atrial enlargement rather than ventricular dilatation.

Ventricular dilation is typically absent in EMF.

RVEMF:

Invariably increased CTR: shape s/o pericardial effusion

RAE: Aneurysmal RA

Oligemic lung fields: characteristic feature

Small hilar vessels

Wide superior mediastinum: Engorged SVC

Pleural effusion: nearly 50 % cases

* Significant right atrial enlargement creates a cardiac silhouette in the shape of the African continent, which is a specific heart shadow sign that has been termed 'the heart of Africa'.

LVEMF:

Slightly enlarged or normal size heart :(Generalized cardiomegaly is unusual).

Evidence of PH with prominent hilar vessels and attenuated peripheral vessels.

LAE: Present but not as marked as RHD

Small aorta

BVEMF:

Finding similar to RVEMF, differentiating point is upper lobe pulmonary veins

In pure right-sided EMF the pulmonary oligemia is striking and the pulmonary veins are inconspicuous. In patients with biventricular EMF, the upper lobe veins are obvious or engorged.

The left ventricle when affected by EMF in biventricular disease is not under as great hemodynamic stress as lone left-sided EMF since it is protected by the low cardiac output of the right side. The functional disturbance on the left side must therefore be relatively severe before decompensation occurs as reflected by pulmonary vein changes.

Electrocardiography

Atrial fibrillation

Seen in 30 – 40 % cases

RVEMF is more frequently associated with AF

Surgical intervention improves prognosis in AF patients

Low QRS voltage

First-degree atrioventricular block in up to 44% of patients

Incomplete right bundle-branch block in up to 30% of patients

Left atrial enlargement

Echocardiography

M Mode features

Dilated atria: Disproportionately enlarged atria in comparison to ventricles is a characteristic feature

Normal dimensions of ventricles are a usual feature.

Thickened LVPW: LVEMF

Thickened IVS: RVEMF

Paradoxical septal motion in RVEMF

2 D Echo features:

Disproportionately dilated atria as compared to ventricles (D/D with DCMP)

RAE with RVEMF; LAE with LVEMF and biatrial dilation in BVEMF. Hugely dilated atria favor EMF to CP

Obliteration of the apex of the involved ventricle: Hallmark of the disease

Thrombi adherent to endocardial surface

Pericardial effusion.

Pleural effusion

Color Doppler features:

MR

TR

E/O pulmonary hypertension

More than moderate PH favors EMF to CP

Diastolic dysfunction with e/o severe restrictive filling pattern with advance disease

Rapid early diastolic filling (E wave) :> 1 m/s

Decreased atrial filling (A wave) :< 0.5 m/s

Reduced deceleration time :< 150 msec

Hepatic / pulmonary vein flow

Systolic forward flow is less than diastolic forward flow

Increased reversal of diastolic flow with inspiration

Decreased flow propagation velocity (Vp): has been demonstrated in a large percentage of patients with EMF. Flow propagation velocity (Vp) is measured as the slope of the first aliasing velocity during early filling, measured from the mitral valve plane to 4 cm distally into LV cavity with color M mode. Normally it is > 50cm/sec.

D/D with other common disease on echocardiography

With dilated cardiomyopathy

Disproportionate atrial enlargement as compared to the corresponding ventricles helps to rule out DCM (Holds true for rheumatic MR or TR also)

Behcet's disease (D/D with RVEMF)

Apical obliteration is due to thrombus

Absence of TR favors Behcet's disease

Huge dilatation of atria does not occur in Behcet's disease

Apical HCM

Apical obliteration occurs during systole only

Apical thrombus

Echocardiographic Thickening of Right Ventricular Anterior Wall; Differential Diagnosis

Primary or secondary pulmonary hypertension

Obstruction to right ventricular outflow

Great arteries transposition with anterior ventricle connected to the aorta

Newborn babies of diabetic mothers

Infiltrative amyloid heart disease

Hypertrophic cardiomyopathy with right ventricular involvement

Tumors of right ventricular anterior wall

Right ventricular endomyocardial fibrosis

Angiography

Traditionally, angiography has been considered as gold standard when making the diagnosis of EMF.

Left and right ventriculography exhibits distortion of chamber morphology by fibrosis and obliteration and variable degrees of mitral and tricuspid regurgitation.

The mushroom sign has been used to describe the shape of the affected ventricle when the apex is obliterated completely by fibrosis.

Electron beam computed tomography scanning

Helps to differentiate CP from EMF.

Typical findings include a band of low attenuation within the endocardium s/o fibrosis.

Obliteration of the apex and inflow tract can also be made out.

Staging

Mocumbi and colleagues provided a set of echocardiographic criteria that is useful in staging the disease, studying its progression, and comparing the results of different epidemiologic studies. In this classification, there are 6 major criteria and 7 minor criteria. The diagnosis is considered when 2 major criteria or 1 major and 2 minor criteria are present. A score has been assigned to each criterion and the severity of the disease is measured by this score; a total score of less than 8 indicates mild endomyocardial fibrosis, a score of 8-15 indicates moderate disease, and a score of more than 15 indicates severe disease.

Major criteria

The following are considered major criteria:

1. Endomyocardial plaques >2 mm in thickness; score: 2
2. Thin (≤1 mm) endomyocardial patches affecting more than one ventricular wall; score: 3
3. Obliteration of the right ventricular or left ventricular apex; score: 4
4. Thrombi or spontaneous contrast without severe ventricular dysfunction; score: 4

5.Retraction of the right ventricular apex (right ventricular apical notch); score: 4

6.Atrioventricular valve dysfunction due to adhesion of the valvular apparatus to the ventricular wall; score: 1–4 (depending on the severity of the regurgitation)

Minor criteria

The following are considered minor criteria:

1. Thin endomyocardial patches localized to 1 ventricular wall; score: 1
2. Restrictive flow pattern across mitral or tricuspid valves; score: 2
3. Pulmonary-valve diastolic opening; score: 2
4. Diffuse thickening of the anterior mitral leaflet; score: 1
5. Enlarged atrium with normal size ventricle; score: 2
6. M-movement of the interventricular septum and flat posterior wall; score: 1
7. Enhanced density of the moderator or other intraventricular bands; score: 1

Natural history

Gupta and colleagues defined the natural history of the disease in Kerala in the late 1980s. Follow up of the initial 200 patients showed a 10 year survival of only 37 per cent. Ascites, atrial fibrillation and New York Heart Association (NYHA) class IV were the poor prognostic indicators. Eighty nine patients, who underwent endocardiectomy with mitral valve replacement, had an actuarial survival of 55 per cent during the same period.

Significant decline in the number of new cases happened in the hospital admissions in Kerala in the subsequent decades. It was related to the change in diet and improved socio-economic status. Cassava and plantain are no longer the staple diet for the Keralites. Natural history in them was more favorable with less than 10 per cent mortality on seven years follow up.

Treatment

Medical Treatment

Symptomatic therapy with

Diuretics has been shown to be useful

Digoxin, afterload reducers and beta-blockers have little role in EMF.

For patients with severe symptoms, consider surgical therapy because the prognosis for these patients with continued medical therapy alone is dismal.

Patients presenting with acute myocarditis, prednisone may be considered as medical therapy.

Role of anticoagulation:

Because the rate of thromboembolism is low among patients with EMF and the patient population affected is not typically compliant with anticoagulation regimens, most authors do not recommend anticoagulant therapy

Surgical Care

Endocardiectomy and AV valve repair or replacement

Palliative procedure

Limitations:

Need for a valve prosthesis,

Cardiac conduction disturbances secondary to endocardiectomy of ventricle, and

The possibility of recurrence of the endocardial fibrosis.

Still it is treatment of choice for this condition because

EMF is characterized by a grave prognosis and medical therapy is ineffective;

EMF is a disease in which only the heart is affected, lesions in other organs being the result of passive congestion;

Systolic performance of the heart is usually only slightly depressed; and surgical procedure is easily performed, so that the mortality is acceptable

The prognosis is poor for patients with diffuse involvement of the heart in EMF, but localized lesions involving the valves are amenable to surgical repair or removal and replacement

Indications:

Advance disease with NYHA class $\geq$ III

Most commonly used approach:

Techniques

Midline thoracotomy

Cardiopulmonary bypass

Transapical or transventricular approach depending on the location of disease (apex or inflow tract)

Endocardiectomy with mitral and/or tricuspid repair or replacement

Endocardiectomy is possible as a well-defined plane of cleavage usually exists between the endocardium and myocardium.

Mortality: high (15 – 20 %)

Is acceptable as

Surgery has a clear benefit on symptoms

Because the myocardium is not usually affected, the severe hemodynamic derangement associated with EMF is relieved with successful resection of the endocardium

Has prognostic benefit in those who survive

Easily performed; hence mortality is not related to surgery

Common postoperative complications include

Low cardiac output,

Heart block, and Ventricular arrhythmias

Indian and Other important Studies

Clinico-pathological evaluation of restrictive cardiomyopathy (endomyocardial fibrosis and idiopathic restrictive cardiomyopathy) in India.

Eur J Heart Fail. 2004 Oct; 6(6):723-9

> Seth S, Thatai D, Sharma S, Chopra P, Talwar KK
>
> N = 52
>
> EMF group = 30
>
> Idiopathic RCMP: 22
>
> EMF group:
>
>> RVEMF: 2
>>
>> BVEMF (Predominant LVEMF): 28

Histomorphologic characteristics of endomyocardial fibrosis: an endomyocardial biopsy study.

Hum Pathol. 1990 Jun;21(6):613-6.

> Chopra P, Narula J, Talwar KK, Kumar V, Bhatia ML.
>
> N = 13
>
> Findings: The endocardium was appreciably thickened due to a cellular hyalinized collagen tissue in all cases. Variable amounts of elastic tissue intimately admixed with fibrous tissue were recognized. A "zonal layering" pattern of the endocardium was absent. Thrombus, inflammatory cells, and granulation tissue at the endomyocardial interphase, and eosinophils within the biopsy were not seen. In addition, lymphomononuclear interstitial inflammatory infiltrates were seen in five cases

Surgical treatment of endomyocardial fibrosis: a new approach

J Am CollCardiol, 1990; 16:1246-1251

> Oliveira et al (Brazil)

Conclusion: Data suggest that resection of endocardial fibrous tissue can be indicated early in the clinical course and performed with preservation of the AV valves.

Clinical course of endomyocardial fibrosis.

Br Heart J. 1989 Dec;62(6):450-4

Gupta PN, Valiathan MS, Balakrishnan KG, Kartha CC, Ghosh MK

N = 145

Percentage survival at the end of 1.0 and 9.5 years was 76.11 and 26.35 respectively

Significant univariate predictors of early mortality

QRS axis more than +90 degrees,

Intraventricular conduction delay (QRS duration > 0.12 s),

Duration of symptoms before presentation,

New York Heart Association functional classes III and IV,

Presence of embolic episodes,

Right atrial mean pressures greater than 20 mm Hg,

Right ventricular end diastolic pressure greater than 20 mm Hg, and

Aortic oxygen saturation less than 85%.

The significant multivariate predictors of mortality were

Cyanosis,

New York Heart Association functional class at first presentation, and

Right atrial mean pressure greater than 20 mm Hg.

Conclusion: The bleak prognosis of endomyocardial fibrosis did not substantially improve despite advances in the medical management of congestive cardiac failure during the period of the study.

Surgical treatment of endomyocardial fibrosis.

Ann Thorac Surg. 1987 Jan; 43(1):68-73.

Valiathan MS, Balakrishnan KG, Sankarkumar R, Kartha CC.

N = 46

Surgery:

Endocardiectomy and

Replacement of tricuspid, mitral, or both atrioventricular valves

The operative mortality within 30 days of the procedure and late mortality during the first two years post operation were 21.7% and 13%

The life table estimate of survival inclusive of operative mortality at two years was 67%

Conclusion: Despite high operative mortality, endocardiectomy with atrioventricular valve replacement is advisable for functionally disabled patients with endomyocardial fibrosis whose prognosis otherwise is dismal

A geochemical basis for endomyocardial fibrosis.

Cardiovasc Res. 1986 Sep; 20(9):679-82

Valiathan MS, Kartha CC, Panday VK, Dang HS, Sunta CM.

Compared with control samples from victims of fatal accidents, an excess of thorium, sodium, and calcium and a deficiency of magnesium were present in samples from patients of EMF.

Conclusion: It is speculated that thorium excess in conjunction with magnesium deficiency may play a role in the causation of tropical endomyocardial fibrosis

Clinical meaning of ascites in patients with endomyocardial fibrosis

Arq Bras Cardiol. 2002 Feb; 78(2):196-9

Barretto AC, Mady C, Oliveira SA, Arteaga E, Dal Bo C, Ramires JA

N = 166

BVEMF: 81 (50.6%)
RVEMF: 28 (17.5%)
LVEMF: 51 (31.8%)

Ascites was present in 67 (41.8%) patients, and right ventricular involvement was present in 59 (88%).

Results;

	With Ascites	Without Ascites
Mortality (%)	49.2	24.7
Associated edema (%)	95	43
Hepatomegaly (cm)	5.8	4.1
RAP (Mean; mm Hg)	19.3	12.0
RVEDP (mm Hg)	18.7	12.9
Duration of illness (yrs)	5.1	3.9
AF (%)	44.7	30.1

CONCLUSION: Ascites was observed in less than 50% of cases of endomyocardial fibrosis and was associated with greater involvement of the right ventricle and with a longer duration of the disease, thus being a characteristic of a worse prognosis.

M-mode echocardiographic features of endomyocardial fibrosis.

Br Heart J. 1982 Sep;48(3):222-8.

George BO, Gaba FE, Talabi AI

N = 21

Features associated with right ventricular endomyocardial fibrosis (n = 13) include:

Exaggerated motion and thickening of the anterior right ventricular wall;

Increased right ventricular end-diastolic dimension; and

Paradoxical septal motion.

Pericardial effusion (an echo-free space behind the posterior left ventricular wall) was shown in three patients.

The tricuspid valve was easily recorded in all.

Features associated with Left ventricular endomyocardial fibrosis (n=6)

Diminished left ventricular end-diastolic dimension.

Three had echo features of pulmonary hypertension (viz reduced e-f slope, absent a wave in sinus rhythm, and systolic notching of the pulmonary valve echogram).

Features associated with BVEMF (n=2):

Fine fluttering of the anterior mitral valve and tricuspid valve echo was observed in two patients (one of whom was in sinus rhythm) with biventricular endomyocardial fibrosis and no angiographic evidence of aortic regurgitation.

Endomyocardial fibrosis in Chandigarh area, India. A study of nine autopsies

Trop Geogr Med. 1977 Dec;29(4):346-52

Datta BN, Babu SK, Khattri HN, Bidwai PS, Wahi PL

These account for nearly 24% of primary cardiomyopathies

BVEMF:	4
LVEMF:	3
RVEMF:	2

Abbreviations

A2:	Aortic component of second heart sound
A2C:	Apical two chamber
A4C:	Apical four chamber
A5C:	Apical five chamber
ACP:	Active constrictive pericarditis
AF:	Atrial Fibrillation
AKT:	Anti Koch's treatment
AR:	Aortic Regurgitation
AV:	Atrioventricular
AV:	Arteriovenous
AV block:	Atrio-ventricular block
AV dissociation:	Atrio-ventricular dissociation
BBB:	Bundle branch block
BNP:	Brain natriuretic peptide
BVEMF:	Bi ventricular endomyocardial fibrosis
BP:	Blood pressure
BT:	Blalock Taussig
CABG:	Coronary artery bypass graft surgery
CAD:	Coronary artery disease
CCF:	Congestive cardiac failure
CCP:	Chronic constrictive pericarditis
CE:	Cardiac enlargement
CHF:	Congestive heart failure
CMP:	Cardiomyopathy
CO:	Cardiac output
COPD:	Chronic obstructive pulmonary disease
CP:	Constrictive pericarditis
CRP:	C reactive protein
CT:	Computed tomography
CTR:	Cardio thoracic ratio
CXR:	Chest X-ray
DCMP:	Dilated cardiomyopathy
D/D:	Differential diagnosis
DT:	Deceleration time
DTI:	Doppler tissue imaging
ECG:	Electrocardiogram
EDD:	End diastolic diameter
EDP:	End diastolic pressure
EF:	Ejection fraction
EMF:	Endomyocardial fibrosis
E/O:	Evidence of
ESC:	European society of cardiology
ESD:	End systolic diameter
ESR:	Erythrocyte sedimentation rate
F/U:	Follow up
FS:	Fractional shortening
HCM:	Hypertrophic cardiomyopathy
IHJ:	Indian Heart Journal

IV:	Intra-venous
IVC:	Inferior vena cava
IVRT:	Isovolumic relaxation time
IVS:	Inter ventricular septum
JVP:	Jugular venous pulse
LA:	Left atrium
LAE:	Left atrial enlargement
LAP:	Left atrial pressure
LAP(m):	Left atrial pressure (mean)
LBBB:	Left bundle branch block
LCC:	Left coronary cusp
LICS:	Left intercostal space
LSB:	Left sterna border
LV:	Left ventricle
LVEMF:	Left ventricular endomyocardial fibrosis
LVEF:	Left ventricular ejection fraction
LVEDP:	Left ventricular end diastolic pressure
LVEDV:	Left ventricular end diastolic volume
LVET:	Left ventricular ejection time
LVF:	Left ventricular failure
LVH:	Left ventricular hypertrophy
LVPW:	Left ventricular posterior wall
MR:	Mitral Regurgitation
MV:	Mitral Valve
MRI:	Magnetic resonance imaging
MVR:	Mitral Valve replacement
NYHA:	New York Heart Association
P2:	Pulmonary component of second heart sound
PA:	Pulmonary artery
PAH:	Pulmonary arterial hypertension
PADP:	Pulmonary artery diastolic pressure
PAP:	Pulmonary artery pressure
PASP:	Pulmonary artery systolic pressure
PAWP:	Pulmonary artery wedge pressure
PCWP:	Pulmonary capillary wedge pressure
PDA:	Patent ductus arteriosus
PEP:	Preejection period
PH:	Pulmonary hypertension
PLAX:	Parasternal long axis
PND:	Paroxysmal nocturnal dyspnea
PS:	Pulmonary stenosis
PSAX:	Parasternal short axis
PSM:	Pansystolic murmur
PV:	Pulmonary valve
PR:	Pulmonary regurgitation
PW:	Posterior wall
RA:	Right atrium
RAE:	Right atrial enlargement
RAP:	Right atrial pressure

Abbreviations

RBBB:	Right bundle branch block
RCMP:	Restrictive cardiomyopathy
RHD:	Rheumatic heart disease
RHF:	Right heart failure
RV:	Right ventricle
RVEF:	Right ventricular ejection fraction
RVEDP:	Right ventricular end diastolic pressure
RVEMF:	Right ventricular endomyocardial fibrosis
RVH:	Right ventricular hypertrophy
RVOT:	Right ventricle outflow tract
RVSP:	Right ventricular systolic pressure
RVVO:	Right ventricular volume overload
S1:	First heart sound
S2:	Second heart sound
S3:	Third heart sound
S4:	Third heart sound
SLE:	Systemic lupus erythematous
SVC:	Superior vena cava
TEE:	Trans esophageal echocardiography
TTE:	Trans thoracic echocardiography
TR:	Tricuspid Regurgitation
TV:	Tricuspid valve
WHO:	World Health Organization

Suggested Reading
Constrictive Pericarditis

1. Wood P (1961) Chronic constrictive pericarditis. Am J Cardiol 7:48–61,
2. Vaitkus PT, Kussmaul WG (1991) Constrictive pericarditis versus restrictive cardiomyopathy: a reappraisal and update of diagnostic criteria. Am Heart J 122:1431–1441
3. Hatle L, Appleton C, Popp R (1989) Differentiation of constrictive pericarditis and restrictive cardiomyopathy by Doppler echocardiography. Circulation 79:357–370
4. Oh JK, Hatle L, Seward JB, et al. (1994) Diagnostic role of Doppler echocardiography in constrictive pericarditis. J Am CollCardiol 23:154–162
5. Rajagopaian N, Garcia MJ, Rodriguez L, et al. (2001) Comparison of new Doppler echocardiographic methods to differentiate constrictive pericardial heart disease and restrictive cardiomyopathy. Am J Cardiol 87:86–94,
6. SpodickDH. Infectious pericarditis. Spodick DH. The pericardium: a comprehensive textbook. New York: Marcel Dekker; 1997. p. 260–290
7. LeWinter MM, Tischler MD. Pericardial diseases. In: Bonow RO, Mann DL, Zipes DP, Libby P, eds. *Braunwald's Heart Disease: A Textbook of Cardiovascular* Medicine. 9th ed. Philadelphia, Pa: Saunders Elsevier; 2011:chap75.
8. Dal-Bianco Jacob, SenguptaPartho, Mookadam Farouk, Chandrasekaran Krishnaswamy, Tajik A Jamil, Khandheria Bijoy: Role of Echocardiography in the Diagnosis of Constrictive Pericarditis. Journal of the American Society of Echocardiography. 2009, 22 (1): 24-33.
9. Little WC, Oh JK. Pericardial diseases. In: Goldman L,Schafer AI, eds. *Cecil Medicine*. 24th ed. Philadelphia, PA: Saunders Elsevier; 2011: chap 77.

Endomyocardial fibrosis

1. Gupta PN, Valiathan MS, Balakrishnan KG, et al. Clinical course of endomyocardial fibrosis. *Br Heart J*. 1989 Dec. 62(6):450-4
2. Mocumbi AO, Ferreira MB, Sidi D, Yacoub MH. A population study of endomyocardial fibrosis in a rural area of Mozambique. *N Engl J Med*. 2008 Jul 3. 359(1):43-9
3. Vijayaraghavan G, Sivasankaran S. Tropical endomyocardial fibrosis in India: a vanishing disease!. *Indian J Med Res*. 2012 Nov. 136(5):729-38
4. Valiathan MS, Balakrishnan KG, Kartha CC. A profile of endomyocardial fibrosis. Indian J Pediatr. 1987;54:229–36
5. Gupta PN, Valiathan MS, Balakrishnan KG, Kartha CC, Ghosh MK. Clinical course of endomyocardial fibrosis. Br Heart J. 1989;62:450–4
6. Marijon E, Hausse AO, Ferreira B.Typical clinical aspect of endomyocardial fibrosis.Int J Cardiol. 2006;112(2):259